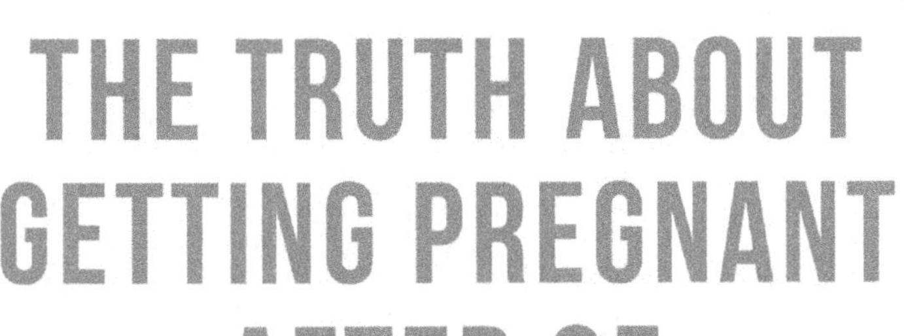

THE TRUTH ABOUT GETTING PREGNANT AFTER 35

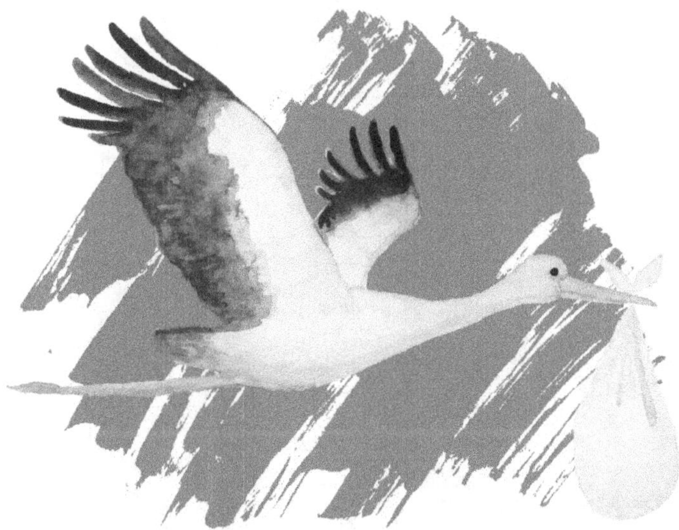

Aurora Brooks

xspurts.com

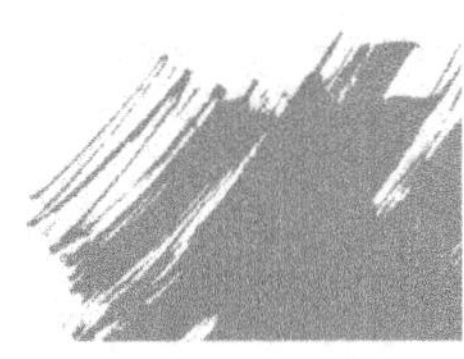

Free Book Offer:
Get How to be a Super Mom For Free

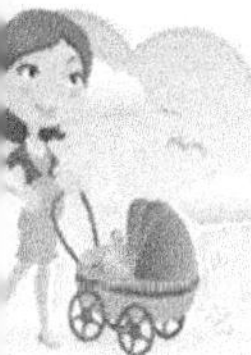

A Short Read is a type of book that is designed to be
read in one quick sitting.

These no fluff books are perfect for people who
want an overview about a subject in a short period o
time.

Table of Contents

<u>**SUPPORTIVE COMMUNITIES**</u>

FREQUENTLY ASKED QUESTIONS

Have Questions / Comments?

Get How To Be A Super Mom 100% FREE

The Truth About Getting Pregnant After 35

e truth about getting pregnant after 35 is a topic that often sparks both curiosity and
ncern among women. Many misconceptions surround the idea of conceiving and
ving a healthy pregnancy at this age, leading to anxiety and confusion. In this
icle, we will explore the realities and debunk the myths surrounding fertility and
gnancy for women over 35 years old.

s important to understand that as women age, their fertility naturally declines. This
cline in fertility is due to various factors, including a decrease in the number and
ality of eggs. While it is still possible for women over 35 to conceive, the chances
getting pregnant naturally decrease compared to younger women.

e relationship between a woman's age and the quality of her eggs is a crucial aspect
consider when trying to conceive after 35. As women age, the number of eggs they
ve in their ovaries decreases, and the remaining eggs may be of lower quality. This
affect the ability to conceive and increase the risk of chromosomal abnormalities
the baby.

arian reserve, which refers to the number and quality of eggs a woman has,
comes a significant factor in fertility after the age of 35. Anti-Mullerian Hormone
MH) levels and antral follicle count are two commonly used indicators to assess
arian reserve and fertility potential. Low AMH levels and a low antral follicle count
y indicate a reduced ovarian reserve, making it more challenging to conceive.

r women who are considering starting a family later in life, egg freezing can be an
tion to preserve fertility. By freezing eggs at a younger age, women can increase
ir chances of getting pregnant in the future, even if their ovarian reserve has
ninished.

wever, it is essential to be aware that getting pregnant after 35 comes with
creased risk factors. Women over 35 have a higher likelihood of experiencing
romosomal abnormalities in their babies, such as Down syndrome. The risk of
veloping gestational diabetes and preeclampsia, a potentially dangerous condition,
o increases with maternal age.

Fortunately, there are various medical interventions available to assist women over in getting pregnant and having a healthy pregnancy. Fertility treatments like in vitro fertilization (IVF) can help overcome fertility challenges and increase the chances of conception. Ovulation induction, which stimulates the ovaries to release eggs, and assisted reproductive technologies like intracytoplasmic sperm injection (ICSI) are other options to consider.

Prenatal screening tests, such as non-invasive prenatal testing (NIPT), play a crucial role in detecting chromosomal abnormalities in older pregnant women. These tests provide valuable information about the baby's health, allowing parents to make informed decisions about their pregnancy.

Before trying to conceive after 35, it is important to prioritize preconception health. Maintaining a balanced diet, engaging in regular exercise, and managing stress are crucial aspects of promoting fertility and a healthy pregnancy. Taking care of one's overall well-being can significantly increase the chances of conceiving and having a successful pregnancy.

Emotionally, trying to conceive and have a baby after the age of 35 can be challenging. Managing stress and seeking support from partners, family, and friends are vital in navigating this journey. Online communities and supportive forums can also provide encouragement and guidance for women trying to conceive later in life.

In some cases, alternative paths to parenthood, such as adoption or surrogacy, may considered for individuals or couples facing difficulties conceiving after 35. Adoption offers a viable option for those who wish to become parents, providing a loving home to a child in need. Surrogacy can also be a possibility for individuals or couples unable to conceive naturally.

Lastly, it is essential to remember that many women have successfully conceived and had healthy pregnancies after the age of 35. Personal experiences and success stories serve as a source of inspiration and hope for those embarking on this journey. With the right support, medical interventions, and a positive mindset, women over 35 can fulfill their dreams of becoming mothers.

Fertility Decline

Understanding the natural decline in fertility as women age is crucial when considering conception after the age of 35. It is a well-known fact that a woman's fertility starts to decline as she gets older, and this decline becomes more significant after the age of 35. This decline occurs due to various factors, including a decrease the number and quality of eggs.

s women age, their ovaries contain fewer eggs, and the remaining eggs may not be s healthy or viable as they were in their younger years. This decline in egg quality an make it more challenging for women over 35 to conceive naturally. Additionally, he chances of chromosomal abnormalities, such as Down syndrome, increase as a oman's age advances.

's important to note that while fertility decline is a natural part of the aging process, does not mean that pregnancy is impossible after the age of 35. Many women uccessfully conceive and have healthy pregnancies in their late thirties and beyond. owever, it is essential to be aware of the potential challenges and take proactive eps to optimize fertility and increase the chances of conception.

Age and Egg Quality

ge plays a significant role in a woman's fertility and the quality of her eggs. As omen age, their egg quantity and quality naturally decline, making it more hallenging to conceive and have a healthy pregnancy. This decline in egg quality is rimarily due to the aging process, which affects the DNA integrity and chromosomal tructure of the eggs.

Vhen a woman is in her 20s, she typically has a higher number of healthy eggs with a wer risk of chromosomal abnormalities. However, as she reaches her mid-30s and eyond, the number of eggs decreases, and the remaining eggs are more likely to have enetic abnormalities. This increases the chances of miscarriage and can make it arder to conceive.

he decline in egg quality can also affect the success of fertility treatments, such as in itro fertilization (IVF). Older women may require more cycles of IVF to achieve a uccessful pregnancy compared to younger women. Additionally, the risk of hromosomal abnormalities, such as Down syndrome, increases with maternal age.

's important for women over 35 who are trying to conceive to be aware of the otential challenges they may face due to age-related decline in egg quality. onsulting with a fertility specialist can provide valuable insights and guidance on the est course of action. They may recommend fertility treatments or other options to nprove the chances of getting pregnant and having a healthy pregnancy.

varian Reserve

he concept of ovarian reserve plays a crucial role in understanding fertility after the ge of 35. Ovarian reserve refers to the quantity and quality of a woman's eggs. As women age, their ovarian reserve naturally declines, which can impact their chances of getting pregnant.

One way to assess ovarian reserve is through the measurement of Anti-Mullerian Hormone (AMH) levels. AMH is produced by the ovaries and can give an indication of the remaining egg supply. Lower levels of AMH may suggest a diminished ovarian reserve, making it more challenging to conceive.

Another indicator of ovarian reserve is the antral follicle count. Antral follicles are small fluid-filled sacs that contain immature eggs. The number of antral follicles visible on an ultrasound can provide insight into a woman's ovarian reserve. A higher antral follicle count is generally associated with a better chance of conceiving.

Understanding ovarian reserve is essential for women over 35 who are trying to conceive. It helps them gauge their fertility potential and make informed decisions about their reproductive options. By consulting with a healthcare professional and monitoring ovarian reserve, women can take proactive steps to optimize their chances of getting pregnant.

AMH Levels

The role of Anti-Mullerian Hormone (AMH) levels in assessing ovarian reserve and fertility potential is a crucial aspect for women over the age of 35 who are trying to conceive. AMH is a hormone produced by the ovarian follicles, and its levels can indicate the quantity and quality of a woman's eggs.

AMH levels are typically measured through a blood test, and they provide valuable information about a woman's ovarian reserve. Ovarian reserve refers to the number of eggs a woman has remaining in her ovaries, and it naturally declines as a woman ages. Low AMH levels may suggest a diminished ovarian reserve, indicating that a woman may have fewer eggs available for fertilization.

Understanding AMH levels can help women over 35 make informed decisions about their fertility options. If AMH levels are low, it may be an indication that fertility treatments such as in vitro fertilization (IVF) or egg freezing could be beneficial. These treatments can help increase the chances of successful conception by using assisted reproductive technologies and preserving eggs for future use.

It's important to note that while AMH levels can provide valuable insights into a woman's fertility potential, they are just one piece of the puzzle. Other factors, such as the quality of eggs and the overall health of the reproductive system, also play a significant role in determining the chances of getting pregnant after 35.

onsulting with a fertility specialist or reproductive endocrinologist can provide a
ore comprehensive understanding of how AMH levels and other factors may impact
rtility. They can help develop a personalized fertility plan and guide women through
e various options available to them.

ntral Follicle Count

ntral follicle count is a crucial factor in assessing a woman's ovarian reserve and
rtility potential. It involves counting the number of small follicles present in the
varies during the early phase of the menstrual cycle. These follicles contain
nmature eggs that have the potential to develop and be released for fertilization.

he antral follicle count is typically determined through ultrasound imaging, which
lows doctors to visualize and count the follicles. A higher antral follicle count is
enerally associated with a higher ovarian reserve, indicating a greater number of
ggs available for fertilization.

his measurement is important for women over 35 who are trying to conceive because
provides valuable information about their fertility status. A lower antral follicle
unt may indicate a diminished ovarian reserve and a decreased likelihood of
iccessful conception.

nowing the antral follicle count can help doctors determine the most appropriate
rtility treatment options for women over 35. It can also help individuals make
formed decisions about their reproductive choices, such as considering egg freezing
pursuing alternative paths to parenthood.

s important to note that while antral follicle count is a useful indicator of ovarian
serve, it is not the only factor that affects fertility. Other factors, such as egg quality
d overall health, also play a significant role in a woman's ability to conceive and
ve a healthy pregnancy.

conclusion, antral follicle count serves as a valuable tool in assessing a woman's
varian reserve and fertility potential. By providing insight into the number of
vailable eggs, it helps individuals and healthcare professionals make informed
cisions regarding fertility treatments and family planning. However, it is essential to
nsider other factors as well and consult with a healthcare provider for personalized
dvice and guidance.

Egg Freezing

Egg freezing, also known as oocyte cryopreservation, is a revolutionary option that allows women to preserve their fertility and increase their chances of getting pregnant in the future. This process involves extracting a woman's eggs and freezing them for later use.

Why would someone consider egg freezing? There are various reasons why women choose this option. Some may want to delay starting a family due to career or personal reasons, while others may be facing medical treatments that could potentially harm their fertility. Whatever the reason may be, egg freezing provides a sense of security and control over one's reproductive future.

The process of egg freezing begins with ovarian stimulation, where the woman takes hormone medications to encourage the production of multiple eggs. These eggs are then retrieved through a minimally invasive procedure called transvaginal ultrasound aspiration. Once retrieved, the eggs are carefully frozen and stored in a specialized facility until the woman is ready to use them.

It is important to note that egg freezing does not guarantee a successful pregnancy in the future. The age at which the eggs were frozen, the quantity and quality of the eggs, and the woman's overall reproductive health all play a role in the success rates of using frozen eggs. However, it does offer a viable option for women who want to preserve their fertility and have the opportunity to conceive later in life.

One of the key benefits of egg freezing is that it allows women to bypass the natural decline in fertility that occurs with age. As women age, the quality and quantity of their eggs diminish, making it more challenging to conceive naturally. By freezing eggs at a younger age, women can preserve their eggs when they are at their healthiest and most viable.

Egg freezing also provides emotional peace of mind for women who may be concerned about their future fertility. It offers a sense of control and empowerment, allowing women to focus on other aspects of their lives without the pressure of starting a family at a specific time.

In conclusion, egg freezing is a valuable option for women who want to preserve their fertility and increase their chances of getting pregnant in the future. It provides a sense of security, control, and peace of mind for those who may be facing various circumstances that could impact their reproductive health. While it is not a guarantee of future pregnancy, it offers hope and opportunity for women to have a family on their own terms.

Increased Risk Factors

women age, there are certain increased risk factors associated with pregnancy after
age of 35. It's important to be aware of these risks and take necessary precautions
ensure a healthy pregnancy. One of the main concerns is the higher likelihood of
romosomal abnormalities in babies born to women over 35. Specifically, the risk of
ving a baby with Down syndrome increases as maternal age advances.

addition to chromosomal abnormalities, there is also an elevated risk of
periencing pregnancy complications after the age of 35. One such complication is
stational diabetes, a condition that affects blood sugar levels during pregnancy.
omen over 35 are more likely to develop gestational diabetes compared to younger
men.

other potential complication is preeclampsia, a condition characterized by high
od pressure and organ damage. Women over 35 are at a higher risk of developing
eclampsia during pregnancy, which can be potentially dangerous for both the
ther and the baby.

important for women over 35 to discuss these increased risk factors with their
althcare provider and receive appropriate prenatal care. Regular check-ups, prenatal
eening tests, and monitoring can help detect and manage these risks effectively. By
ing proactive and taking necessary precautions, women can increase their chances
having a healthy pregnancy and a successful outcome.

wn Syndrome

wn Syndrome is a chromosomal disorder that occurs when there is an extra copy of
romosome 21. It is one of the most common genetic conditions and is associated
th intellectual disabilities and certain physical characteristics. While Down
ndrome can occur in babies born to women of any age, the risk increases as
ternal age advances, particularly after the age of 35.

search has shown that the chances of having a baby with Down Syndrome increase
nificantly for women over 35. This is because as women age, the quality of their
gs decreases, and there is a higher likelihood of chromosomal abnormalities
curring during fertilization. The risk of Down Syndrome at age 35 is approximately
n 350, while at age 40, it increases to 1 in 100.

important for women over 35 to be aware of this increased risk and to consider
enatal screening tests to assess the likelihood of their baby having Down Syndrome.
ese tests can include non-invasive prenatal testing (NIPT), which analyzes the fetal

DNA in the mother's blood, or diagnostic procedures such as chorionic villus
sampling (CVS) or amniocentesis.

While the risk of having a baby with Down Syndrome may be higher for women ov
35, it is essential to remember that the majority of babies born to older mothers are
still typically healthy. It is a personal decision whether to pursue further testing or n
and it is important to consult with healthcare professionals to fully understand the
options and implications.

Gestational Diabetes

Gestational diabetes is a condition that affects pregnant women, and it is more likely
to occur in women who are over the age of 35. This condition is characterized by hi
blood sugar levels that occur during pregnancy, and it usually resolves after giving
birth. However, it is important to recognize and manage gestational diabetes as it ca
have potential risks for both the mother and the baby.

When a woman is pregnant, her body goes through hormonal changes that can affec
how insulin, a hormone that regulates blood sugar, works. In some cases, the body
may not be able to produce enough insulin to effectively manage the increased bloo
sugar levels during pregnancy. This leads to gestational diabetes.

Women who are over the age of 35 are at a higher risk of developing gestational
diabetes due to several factors. Firstly, as women age, their bodies may become less
sensitive to insulin, making it harder for the body to regulate blood sugar levels.
Additionally, women who are overweight or have a family history of diabetes are al
more prone to developing gestational diabetes.

It is important to monitor and manage gestational diabetes to prevent complications
during pregnancy. Women with gestational diabetes may need to make certain
lifestyle changes, such as following a healthy diet and engaging in regular physical
activity. In some cases, medication or insulin injections may be necessary to control
blood sugar levels.

Gestational diabetes can have potential risks for both the mother and the baby. If lei
unmanaged, it can increase the risk of high blood pressure, preeclampsia, and the no
for a cesarean delivery. It can also lead to excessive birth weight, which can increas
the risk of complications during delivery. Furthermore, babies born to mothers with
gestational diabetes may be at a higher risk of developing type 2 diabetes later in lif

Regular prenatal care and monitoring are essential for women over the age of 35 to
detect and manage gestational diabetes. Healthcare providers may recommend regu

lood sugar testing, as well as additional ultrasounds to monitor the baby's growth and
evelopment.

1 conclusion, women over the age of 35 have a higher likelihood of developing
estational diabetes during pregnancy. It is important for expectant mothers in this age
roup to be aware of the risks and to work closely with their healthcare providers to
1anage and monitor their blood sugar levels. By taking proactive steps to control
estational diabetes, women can have a healthier pregnancy and reduce the potential
sks for both themselves and their babies.

reeclampsia

reeclampsia is a serious condition that can occur during pregnancy, and women over
1e age of 35 are at an increased risk. This condition is characterized by high blood
ressure and damage to organs such as the liver and kidneys. It can also affect the
lacenta, which can lead to complications for both the mother and the baby.

'he exact cause of preeclampsia is not fully understood, but it is believed to be related
) problems with the placenta. Women over 35 may be more susceptible to this
ondition due to age-related changes in blood vessels and the placenta. Additionally,
romen who have pre-existing conditions such as high blood pressure or diabetes are
t an even higher risk.

: is important for women over 35 to be aware of the signs and symptoms of
reeclampsia, as early detection and treatment can greatly reduce the risk of
omplications. Some common symptoms include high blood pressure, swelling in the
ands and face, headaches, and changes in vision. Regular prenatal check-ups and
1onitoring of blood pressure and urine protein levels are essential for early detection.

preeclampsia is diagnosed, medical interventions may be necessary to manage the
ondition and protect the health of both the mother and the baby. Treatment options
1ay include medication to lower blood pressure, bed rest, and close monitoring of the
aby's growth and well-being. In severe cases, early delivery of the baby may be
ecessary to prevent further complications.

is important for women over 35 to work closely with their healthcare provider
1roughout their pregnancy to monitor for signs of preeclampsia and take any
ecessary precautions. Maintaining a healthy lifestyle, including regular exercise, a
alanced diet, and managing stress, can also help reduce the risk of developing
reeclampsia.

In conclusion, preeclampsia is a serious condition that can occur during pregnancy, and women over the age of 35 are at an increased risk. It is important for women in this age group to be aware of the signs and symptoms and to seek medical attention if any concerns arise. With proper monitoring and medical interventions, the risk of complications can be minimized, and a healthy pregnancy can still be achieved.

Medical Interventions

Medical interventions play a crucial role in assisting women over the age of 35 in their journey to conceive and have a healthy pregnancy. As fertility declines with age, these interventions can help overcome challenges and increase the chances of successful conception.

One of the most common medical interventions is fertility treatments, such as in vitro fertilization (IVF). IVF involves the retrieval of eggs from the ovaries, fertilizing them with sperm in a laboratory, and then transferring the embryos into the uterus. This procedure can bypass age-related fertility issues and increase the likelihood of pregnancy.

In addition to IVF, ovulation induction is another medical intervention that can assist women over 35 in getting pregnant. This process involves the use of medications, such as Clomid or letrozole, to stimulate the ovaries and promote the release of eggs. Ovulation induction can help regulate the menstrual cycle and improve the chances of conception.

Assisted reproductive technologies, such as intracytoplasmic sperm injection (ICSI), are also available to overcome fertility challenges. ICSI involves injecting a single sperm directly into an egg, increasing the chances of fertilization. This technique can be particularly helpful for couples dealing with male factor infertility.

Prenatal screening tests, such as non-invasive prenatal testing (NIPT), are essential for older pregnant women. These tests can detect chromosomal abnormalities, such as Down syndrome, in the fetus. Early detection allows for informed decision-making and appropriate medical care throughout the pregnancy.

It is important to consult with a fertility specialist or reproductive endocrinologist to explore the various medical interventions available and determine the most suitable approach for individual circumstances. These interventions, combined with proper preconception care and support, can greatly increase the chances of achieving a successful pregnancy after the age of 35.

Fertility Treatments

Fertility treatments offer hope to women over 35 who are struggling to conceive naturally. One of the most well-known and widely used fertility treatments is in vitro fertilization (IVF). IVF involves the retrieval of eggs from the woman's ovaries and the fertilization of these eggs with sperm in a laboratory setting. The resulting embryos are then transferred back into the woman's uterus, where they have the potential to implant and develop into a pregnancy.

IVF can be a suitable option for women over 35 who have been unsuccessful in conceiving through other means. It allows for the direct manipulation of eggs and sperm, increasing the chances of successful fertilization and implantation. Additionally, IVF can also help overcome certain fertility challenges, such as blocked fallopian tubes or low sperm count.

However, it's important to note that IVF may not be the right choice for everyone. The process can be physically and emotionally demanding, and success rates can vary depending on factors such as age and overall health. It's crucial to consult with a fertility specialist to determine the most appropriate treatment plan based on individual circumstances.

Ovulation Induction

Ovulation induction is a medical intervention that can assist women over 35 in getting pregnant. It involves stimulating the ovaries to produce multiple eggs, increasing the chances of successful conception. This process is often recommended for women who have irregular or infrequent menstrual cycles, or those who are not ovulating regularly.

There are several methods of ovulation induction, but the most common approach is through the use of fertility medications. These medications, such as Clomid or Letrozole, work by stimulating the production of follicle-stimulating hormone (FSH) in the body. FSH is responsible for the growth and development of ovarian follicles, which contain the eggs.

Once the follicles have reached a certain size, a trigger shot of human chorionic gonadotropin (hCG) is administered to induce ovulation. This triggers the release of the mature eggs from the follicles, making them available for fertilization. Ovulation induction is often combined with timed intercourse or intrauterine insemination (IUI) to maximize the chances of conception.

This process plays a crucial role in assisting women over 35 in getting pregnant because it helps overcome the age-related decline in fertility. As women age, the number and quality of their eggs decrease, making it more challenging to conceive naturally. Ovulation induction increases the number of eggs available for fertilization increasing the likelihood of successful conception and pregnancy.

Assisted Reproductive Technologies

Assisted Reproductive Technologies (ART) have revolutionized the field of fertility treatment, offering hope to women over 35 who are facing challenges in conceiving. One such technique is intracytoplasmic sperm injection (ICSI), which has proven to be a successful method in overcoming fertility obstacles.

ICSI involves the direct injection of a single sperm into an egg, bypassing any potential barriers that may exist. This procedure is particularly beneficial for couples where the male partner has low sperm count or poor sperm quality. By directly injecting a healthy sperm into the egg, the chances of fertilization and successful implantation are significantly increased.

ICSI is performed as part of an in vitro fertilization (IVF) cycle. During the IVF process, the woman's eggs are retrieved and then carefully examined under a microscope. The embryologist selects the healthiest and most viable eggs for fertilization. With ICSI, a single sperm is carefully injected into each selected egg, allowing for precise control and increasing the chances of successful fertilization.

ICSI has proven to be a game-changer for couples struggling with fertility issues after the age of 35. It offers a ray of hope by providing a solution to overcome male factor infertility or other obstacles that may hinder natural conception. With advancements in ART, such as ICSI, the dream of starting a family can become a reality for many couples facing fertility challenges.

Prenatal Screening

Prenatal screening is a crucial aspect of prenatal care for women over the age of 35. As women age, the risk of chromosomal abnormalities in their unborn babies increases. Prenatal screening tests, such as non-invasive prenatal testing (NIPT), play a significant role in detecting these abnormalities early on.

NIPT is a non-invasive procedure that involves a simple blood test. It screens for common chromosomal conditions, such as Down syndrome, trisomy 18, and trisomy 13. Unlike invasive procedures like amniocentesis or chorionic villus sampling (CVS), NIPT carries no risk of miscarriage.

ring NIPT, a small sample of the mother's blood is taken and analyzed for fetal
JA. The test can accurately determine the risk of chromosomal abnormalities in the
oy as early as 10 weeks into the pregnancy. It is a highly reliable screening method,
:h a low false-positive rate.

r women over 35, prenatal screening tests like NIPT provide valuable information
out the health of their unborn baby. If the results indicate a higher risk of
romosomal abnormalities, further diagnostic tests may be recommended to confirm
: findings.

important to note that prenatal screening tests do not provide a definitive
gnosis. They only indicate the likelihood of a chromosomal abnormality. In the
ent of a positive result, genetic counseling and additional diagnostic tests, such as
niocentesis or CVS, may be recommended to provide a conclusive diagnosis.

erall, prenatal screening tests like NIPT are essential tools in the care of older
egnant women. They offer peace of mind and enable healthcare providers to provide
propriate support and interventions if necessary. It's crucial for women over 35 to
cuss these screening options with their healthcare providers and make informed
cisions about their prenatal care.

Preconception Health

nen it comes to getting pregnant after the age of 35, maintaining good overall health
d adopting healthy lifestyle choices become even more crucial. Preconception
alth plays a significant role in increasing the chances of a successful pregnancy and
suring the well-being of both the mother and the baby.

e of the key aspects of preconception health is optimal nutrition. A balanced diet
t includes a variety of fruits, vegetables, whole grains, lean proteins, and healthy
s provides the necessary nutrients for reproductive health. It is also important to
y hydrated and limit the consumption of processed foods, sugary drinks, and
feine.

gular exercise is another important factor in preconception health. Engaging in
oderate physical activity, such as walking, swimming, or yoga, not only helps
intain a healthy weight but also improves fertility. Exercise promotes proper blood
culation, reduces stress, and boosts overall well-being, all of which are beneficial
women trying to conceive after 35.

addition to nutrition and exercise, it is crucial to address any underlying health
nditions before attempting to conceive. This may involve consulting with healthcare

professionals to manage chronic conditions like diabetes or hypertension. It is also important to review any medications being taken and discuss their potential impact fertility and pregnancy.

Taking care of one's mental and emotional well-being is equally important during the preconception period. Stress management techniques, such as meditation, deep breathing exercises, or engaging in hobbies, can help alleviate the emotional toll of trying to get pregnant after 35. Building a strong support system with partners, family and friends can provide the necessary emotional support and guidance throughout the journey.

In summary, preconception health plays a vital role in increasing the chances of a successful pregnancy for women over 35. By maintaining good overall health, adopting a healthy lifestyle, and addressing any underlying health conditions, women can optimize their fertility and create the best possible environment for a healthy pregnancy and baby.

Optimal Nutrition

Optimal nutrition plays a crucial role in promoting fertility and ensuring a healthy pregnancy for women over 35. As women age, their bodies undergo natural changes that can impact their ability to conceive and maintain a pregnancy. By focusing on a balanced diet and proper nutrition, women can support their reproductive health and increase their chances of getting pregnant.

A balanced diet for women over 35 should include a variety of nutrient-rich foods that provide essential vitamins and minerals. This includes consuming plenty of fruits, vegetables, whole grains, lean proteins, and healthy fats. These foods provide the necessary nutrients to support reproductive function and hormone balance.

In addition to a balanced diet, it is important for women over 35 to pay attention to specific nutrients that are particularly important for fertility and pregnancy. These include folic acid, iron, calcium, omega-3 fatty acids, and antioxidants. Folic acid, for example, is crucial for preventing birth defects and should be taken as a supplement before and during pregnancy.

Proper hydration is also essential for maintaining optimal fertility and a healthy pregnancy. Drinking an adequate amount of water helps to support overall health and ensures that the body is functioning optimally. It is recommended to drink at least 8 cups of water per day.

is worth noting that individual nutritional needs may vary, and it is always a good
idea to consult with a healthcare professional or a registered dietitian for personalized
advice. They can help create a tailored nutrition plan that takes into account any
specific dietary requirements or health concerns.

Overall, maintaining a balanced diet and focusing on proper nutrition can significantly
improve fertility and increase the chances of having a healthy pregnancy for women
over 35. By nourishing the body with the right nutrients, women can support their
reproductive health and increase their chances of conceiving and having a successful
pregnancy.

Regular Exercise

Regular exercise plays a crucial role in improving fertility and reducing pregnancy
complications for women over 35. Engaging in physical activity not only enhances
overall health but also increases the chances of conception and a healthy pregnancy.
Let's explore the benefits of regular exercise for women in this age group.

1. Enhanced Fertility: Regular exercise can improve fertility by regulating hormonal
levels, increasing blood flow to the reproductive organs, and promoting healthy
ovulation. It can also help maintain a healthy body weight, which is essential for
optimal fertility.

2. Reduced Risk of Pregnancy Complications: Women over 35 are at a higher risk of
developing pregnancy complications such as gestational diabetes and preeclampsia.
However, regular exercise can help reduce these risks by improving blood sugar
control, maintaining healthy blood pressure levels, and strengthening the
cardiovascular system.

3. Improved Mental Well-being: Trying to conceive and undergoing fertility
treatments can be emotionally challenging for women over 35. Regular exercise acts
as a natural stress reliever, releasing endorphins that boost mood and reduce anxiety
and depression. It also provides a sense of empowerment and control over one's body
and fertility journey.

4. Healthy Weight Management: Maintaining a healthy weight is crucial for fertility
and a successful pregnancy. Regular exercise helps burn calories, build lean muscle
mass, and improve metabolism, aiding in weight management. It also promotes
healthy body composition and reduces the risk of obesity-related complications during
pregnancy.

5. Increased Energy Levels: Pregnancy can be physically demanding, especially for women over 35. Regular exercise helps improve stamina and energy levels, making it easier to cope with the physical demands of pregnancy and childbirth.

To incorporate regular exercise into your routine, consider activities such as brisk walking, swimming, yoga, or low-impact aerobics. It's important to consult with your healthcare provider before starting any exercise program, especially if you have any underlying health conditions or are undergoing fertility treatments.

Remember, moderation is key. Aim for at least 150 minutes of moderate-intensity exercise per week, spread across several days. Listen to your body and avoid overexertion or high-impact activities that may pose a risk to your health or pregnancy.

By prioritizing regular exercise, women over 35 can improve their fertility, reduce pregnancy complications, and enhance their overall well-being. It's never too late to start taking care of your health and increasing your chances of a successful pregnancy

Emotional Considerations

Trying to conceive and have a baby after the age of 35 can bring about a range of emotional considerations and potential challenges. It's important to address these aspects and understand the impact they can have on your journey towards parenthood

One of the main emotional considerations is the pressure and stress that can come with trying to conceive at an older age. As time goes on, the fear of not being able to get pregnant or experiencing fertility issues can become overwhelming. It's crucial to find effective stress management techniques to cope with these emotions and maintain a positive mindset.

Building a strong support system is also essential during this time. Having a partner, family, and friends who understand and support your desire to have a baby can make significant difference. They can provide emotional support, offer advice, and be there for you during the highs and lows of your journey.

Additionally, it can be helpful to connect with others who are going through a similar experience. Supportive communities and online forums can provide a sense of belonging and offer a space to share experiences, ask questions, and receive encouragement. Knowing that you're not alone in your journey can provide a sense of comfort and reassurance.

s important to acknowledge that trying to conceive after 35 may come with its own
unique challenges. However, with the right emotional support, stress management
techniques, and a positive mindset, it is possible to navigate these challenges and
fulfill your dream of becoming a parent.

Stress Management

Trying to get pregnant after the age of 35 can be emotionally challenging, as the
pressure to conceive can often lead to increased stress levels. However, effective
stress management techniques can help women cope with the emotional toll of trying
to conceive. Here are some strategies that can be beneficial:

- **1. Mindfulness and Meditation:** Practicing mindfulness and meditation can
  help reduce stress and promote relaxation. Taking a few minutes each day to
  focus on your breath and be present in the moment can have a calming effect
  on the mind and body.
- **2. Exercise:** Engaging in regular physical activity can release endorphins,
  which are natural mood boosters. Whether it's going for a walk, practicing
  yoga, or participating in a fitness class, finding an exercise routine that you
  enjoy can help alleviate stress.
- **3. Support Network:** Surrounding yourself with a strong support network of
  friends, family, and other women going through similar experiences can
  provide a sense of comfort and understanding. Sharing your feelings and
  concerns with others who can empathize can help alleviate stress.
- **4. Relaxation Techniques:** Trying relaxation techniques such as deep
  breathing exercises, progressive muscle relaxation, or taking warm baths can
  help calm the mind and body. Finding activities that help you unwind and relax
  can be beneficial in managing stress.
- **5. Self-Care:** Prioritizing self-care is essential when dealing with the emotional
  challenges of trying to conceive. Taking time for yourself, engaging in
  activities that bring you joy, and practicing self-compassion can help reduce
  stress levels.

Remember, stress can negatively impact fertility, so it's important to find healthy
ways to manage and cope with stress during this journey. By incorporating these
stress management techniques into your daily routine, you can create a more positive
and balanced mindset while trying to get pregnant after 35.

Support Systems

The journey of getting pregnant after the age of 35 can be filled with various
challenges and uncertainties. It is during this time that having a strong support system

becomes crucial. Support systems, including partners, family, and friends, play a vital role in providing emotional, physical, and practical support throughout the process.

Partners are often the first line of support for women trying to conceive after 35. They can offer understanding, empathy, and encouragement during the ups and downs of the journey. It is important for partners to be involved and informed about the process as it can help strengthen the bond and create a sense of shared responsibility.

Family members can also provide invaluable support during this time. They can offer assistance with childcare, household chores, and provide a listening ear when needed. Family support can help alleviate some of the stress and pressure associated with trying to conceive and having a healthy pregnancy.

Friends can play a significant role in providing emotional support and understanding. They can offer a safe space to talk about fears, frustrations, and hopes. Friends who have gone through a similar journey can provide valuable insights and advice, creating a sense of camaraderie and shared experiences.

Aside from personal support, joining support groups or online communities can also be beneficial. These platforms allow individuals to connect with others who are going through similar experiences. They provide a space for sharing stories, asking questions, and receiving support from individuals who truly understand the challenges and emotions involved.

In conclusion, having a strong support system is crucial for women trying to conceive after the age of 35. Partners, family, friends, and supportive communities can provide the emotional, physical, and practical support needed during this journey. They offer encouragement, understanding, and guidance, making the process a little easier and less daunting. Remember, you don't have to go through it alone.

Alternative Paths to Parenthood

Alternative Paths to Parenthood

For those who face difficulties conceiving after 35, there are alternative paths to parenthood that can be considered. Adoption and surrogacy are two options that provide hope and the opportunity to fulfill the dream of becoming a parent.

Adoption:

Adoption is a viable path to parenthood for individuals or couples over 35. It offers the chance to provide a loving home to a child in need and create a family through a al process. There are various options available for adoption, including domestic option, international adoption, and foster care adoption. Each option has its own ique requirements and considerations, but they all offer the possibility of periencing the joys of parenthood.

rrogacy:

rrogacy is another alternative option for individuals or couples unable to conceive er 35. It involves a woman carrying and giving birth to a child on behalf of another rson or couple. There are different types of surrogacy, including traditional rogacy and gestational surrogacy. In traditional surrogacy, the surrogate mother es her own egg, while in gestational surrogacy, the embryo is created using the ended parent's or a donor's egg and sperm. Surrogacy can be a complex process, but offers the hope of having a biological connection to the child and experiencing the of parenthood.

hen considering alternative paths to parenthood, it is important to thoroughly earch and understand the legal and emotional aspects of adoption and surrogacy. nsulting with professionals and seeking support from others who have gone ough similar experiences can provide valuable guidance and reassurance.

member, parenthood can be achieved through various paths, and age should not be arrier to fulfilling the desire to have a child. With determination, support, and the ploration of alternative options, the dream of becoming a parent can become a lity.

option

option can be a wonderful and fulfilling option for individuals or couples over the e of 35 who are unable to conceive. It provides a viable path to parenthood and the portunity to create a loving family. The process of adoption involves several steps, luding evaluation, preparation, and matching with a child.

hen considering adoption, it is important to research and understand the different es of adoption available. These options include domestic adoption, international option, and foster care adoption. Each type has its own unique requirements and siderations.

domestic adoption, individuals or couples work with adoption agencies or attorneys adopt a child within their own country. This process often involves home studies, ckground checks, and interviews to assess the prospective adoptive parents' tability and readiness to provide a loving and stable home.

International adoption involves adopting a child from another country. This process typically includes working with an adoption agency that specializes in international adoption. Prospective adoptive parents must meet the requirements set by both their home country and the country they are adopting from. These requirements may include age limits, marital status, and financial stability.

Foster care adoption is another option for individuals or couples over 35. It involves adopting a child who is in the foster care system. Prospective adoptive parents must go through a rigorous screening process, including home studies and training, to ensure they can provide a safe and nurturing environment for the child.

Once the adoption process is complete, individuals or couples over 35 can experience the joy of parenthood through adoption. It is important to note that the age of the prospective adoptive parents may be a factor in the adoption process, as some countries or agencies may have age restrictions or preferences.

Adoption offers a unique and rewarding path to parenthood for individuals or couples over 35. It provides the opportunity to give a child a loving and stable home, while fulfilling the desire to become parents. It is important to consult with adoption professionals and do thorough research to understand the process and options available.

Surrogacy

Surrogacy:

Surrogacy is a viable alternative option for individuals or couples who are unable to conceive after the age of 35. It involves a woman, known as the surrogate, carrying and giving birth to a baby on behalf of the intended parents. This arrangement allows individuals or couples to experience the joys of parenthood despite facing challenges with conception.

Types of Surrogacy:

There are two main types of surrogacy: traditional surrogacy and gestational surrogacy. Traditional surrogacy involves the surrogate using her own eggs to conceive the baby, making her the biological mother. Gestational surrogacy, on the other hand, involves the use of in vitro fertilization (IVF) to implant an embryo created from the intended parents' eggs and sperm into the surrogate's uterus. In this case, the surrogate is not genetically related to the baby.

The Process:

urrogacy involves a complex and highly regulated process. It typically begins with
ie intended parents finding a suitable surrogate through a surrogacy agency or a
nown surrogate. Legal agreements are then drafted to outline the rights and
:sponsibilities of all parties involved.

)nce the legalities are sorted, the medical process begins. The intended mother or a
onor undergoes ovarian stimulation to produce multiple eggs, which are then
:rtilized with the intended father's sperm in a laboratory. The resulting embryos are
ansferred to the surrogate's uterus, and if successful, pregnancy occurs.

Benefits and Considerations:

urrogacy offers several benefits for individuals or couples unable to conceive after
ie age of 35. It provides them with the opportunity to have a biological child and
xperience the joys of parenthood. Surrogacy also allows individuals or couples to
iaintain a genetic connection to their child, which can be important for some.

Iowever, it's important to consider the emotional and financial aspects of surrogacy.
'he process can be emotionally challenging, as it involves relying on another woman
） carry and give birth to the baby. Additionally, surrogacy can be expensive, with
osts varying depending on factors such as the location and the specific arrangements
iade.

Legal and Ethical Considerations:

urrogacy laws and regulations vary from country to country and even within
ifferent states or regions. It's crucial to thoroughly research and understand the legal
nd ethical aspects of surrogacy in the intended location. Working with a reputable
irrogacy agency can provide guidance and support throughout the process.

Conclusion:

urrogacy offers hope and an alternative path to parenthood for individuals or couples
iable to conceive after the age of 35. It allows them to fulfill their dreams of having
 child and experiencing the joys of raising a family. By understanding the process,
onsidering the emotional and financial aspects, and navigating the legal and ethical
onsiderations, individuals or couples can make informed decisions about pursuing
irrogacy as an option for building their family.

Success Stories

Success stories of women who successfully conceived and had healthy pregnancies after the age of 35 serve as a source of inspiration and hope for those who may be facing challenges in their journey to parenthood. These stories demonstrate that age does not have to be a barrier to starting or expanding a family.

One such success story is Sarah, who at the age of 38, decided to pursue her dream of becoming a mother. Despite initial concerns about her age and fertility, Sarah remained optimistic and sought the guidance of a fertility specialist. Through assisted reproductive technologies, Sarah was able to conceive and went on to have a healthy pregnancy, giving birth to a beautiful baby girl.

Another inspiring story is that of Lisa, who at the age of 40, decided to explore the option of adoption after struggling with infertility. After a lengthy and emotional process, Lisa and her husband were matched with a birth mother and welcomed their son into their family. Through the journey of adoption, Lisa found a sense of fulfillment and joy in becoming a mother, regardless of her age.

These success stories highlight the resilience and determination of women who refuse to let age define their ability to have a family. They serve as a reminder that there are alternative paths to parenthood, such as adoption or surrogacy, for those who may face difficulties conceiving naturally after 35.

In addition to the personal experiences of these women, supportive communities and online forums play a crucial role in providing encouragement and guidance for those trying to conceive after 35. These communities provide a safe space for individuals to share their stories, seek advice, and find solace in knowing they are not alone in their journey.

Ultimately, the success stories of women who have overcome challenges and achieve their dreams of becoming mothers after 35 serve as a beacon of hope for others facing similar circumstances. They remind us that with perseverance, support, and the right medical interventions, it is possible to have a healthy pregnancy and bring a child into the world, regardless of age.

Personal Experiences

Personal Experiences

It is important to recognize and celebrate the personal journeys of women who have successfully conceived and had healthy pregnancies after the age of 35. These stories serve as a source of inspiration and hope for those who may be facing challenges in their own fertility journey.

ne such story is that of Sarah, who at the age of 37, decided to pursue her dream of
:coming a mother. Despite initial concerns about her age and fertility, Sarah
mained optimistic and sought the guidance of fertility specialists. Through the
ocess of in vitro fertilization (IVF), Sarah was able to conceive and carry a healthy
egnancy to term. Today, she is the proud mother of a beautiful baby girl and serves
a reminder that age should not be a deterrent to fulfilling one's desire for
otherhood.

nother inspiring story is that of Lisa, who at the age of 40, faced multiple
iscarriages and fertility setbacks. Determined to never give up on her dream of
ving a child, Lisa explored alternative options and decided to pursue adoption. After
lengthy and emotional process, Lisa and her husband were matched with a baby boy
ho brought immense joy and love into their lives. Lisa's story showcases the
silience and strength of women who refuse to let age define their journey to
arenthood.

hese personal experiences highlight the triumphs and challenges that women may
ncounter when trying to conceive after the age of 35. They demonstrate that with
erseverance, support, and the right medical interventions, it is possible to overcome
ostacles and achieve the dream of becoming a mother. It is important for women in
milar situations to seek support from their loved ones and connect with supportive
ommunities and online forums where they can find encouragement, guidance, and
ared experiences.

pportive Communities

apportive communities and online forums play a crucial role in providing
ncouragement and guidance for women who are trying to conceive after the age of
5. These communities serve as a valuable resource for women who may be facing
allenges or seeking information about fertility, pregnancy, and motherhood.

ne of the main benefits of joining a supportive community is the opportunity to
onnect with other women who are going through similar experiences. Sharing
ories, advice, and concerns with others who understand the unique challenges of
ying to conceive later in life can be incredibly comforting and empowering. These
ommunities provide a safe space for women to express their feelings, ask questions,
id receive support from others who can relate.

nline forums also offer a wealth of information and resources. Women can find
xpert advice, research studies, and articles on topics such as fertility treatments,
enatal care, and preconception health. These resources can help women make
formed decisions and navigate the complexities of trying to conceive after 35.

Furthermore, supportive communities often organize meetups, events, and workshop
where women can connect in person. These gatherings provide an opportunity to for
deeper connections, share personal experiences, and build a strong support network.
can be incredibly empowering to surround oneself with like-minded individuals who
understand the journey and can offer guidance and encouragement along the way.

In conclusion, supportive communities and online forums play a vital role in
providing encouragement and guidance for women trying to conceive after the age o
35. These communities offer a safe space for women to connect, share experiences,
and access valuable resources. By joining these communities, women can find the
support they need to navigate the challenges and uncertainties of trying to conceive
later in life.

Frequently Asked Questions

- **1. Can women over 35 still get pregnant?**

  Yes, women over 35 can still get pregnant. However, it is important to
  understand that fertility declines as women age, and the chances of conceiving
  naturally may decrease. Seeking medical advice and exploring fertility
  treatments can increase the chances of getting pregnant.

- **2. Does age affect the quality of eggs?**

  Yes, age can affect the quality of eggs. As women get older, the number of
  eggs in their ovaries decreases, and the remaining eggs may have a higher risk
  of chromosomal abnormalities. This can impact the chances of successful
  conception and increase the risk of certain pregnancy complications.

- **3. What is ovarian reserve?**

  Ovarian reserve refers to the number and quality of eggs a woman has in her
  ovaries. It is an important factor in determining fertility potential. As women
  age, their ovarian reserve naturally declines, which can make it more
  challenging to conceive.

- **4. How can ovarian reserve be assessed?**

  Ovarian reserve can be assessed through tests such as Anti-Mullerian Hormor
  (AMH) levels and antral follicle count. These tests provide insights into the
  quantity and quality of eggs remaining in the ovaries, helping to evaluate
  fertility potential.

5. Is egg freezing a viable option?

Yes, egg freezing can be a viable option for women over 35 who want to preserve their fertility. By freezing eggs at a younger age, women can increase their chances of successful conception in the future.

6. Are there increased risks associated with pregnancy after 35?

Yes, there are increased risks associated with pregnancy after 35. These include a higher likelihood of chromosomal abnormalities such as Down syndrome, as well as an elevated risk of developing gestational diabetes and preeclampsia.

7. What medical interventions are available?

There are various medical interventions available to assist women over 35 in getting pregnant and having a healthy pregnancy. Fertility treatments like in vitro fertilization (IVF) and ovulation induction can help overcome fertility challenges. Prenatal screening tests can also detect chromosomal abnormalities.

8. How important is preconception health?

Preconception health is crucial for women over 35 who are trying to conceive. Maintaining a balanced diet, engaging in regular exercise, and managing stress can improve fertility and reduce the risk of pregnancy complications.

9. What emotional considerations should be taken into account?

Trying to conceive and having a baby after the age of 35 can bring emotional challenges. Effective stress management techniques and having a strong support system can help cope with the emotional toll of the journey.

10. Are there alternative paths to parenthood?

Yes, there are alternative paths to parenthood for individuals or couples unable to conceive after 35. Adoption and surrogacy are options that can help fulfill the desire to become parents.

11. Are there success stories of women conceiving after 35?

Absolutely! Many women have successfully conceived and had healthy pregnancies after the age of 35. Hearing personal experiences and being part of supportive communities can provide encouragement and guidance throughout the journey.

Have Questions / Comments?

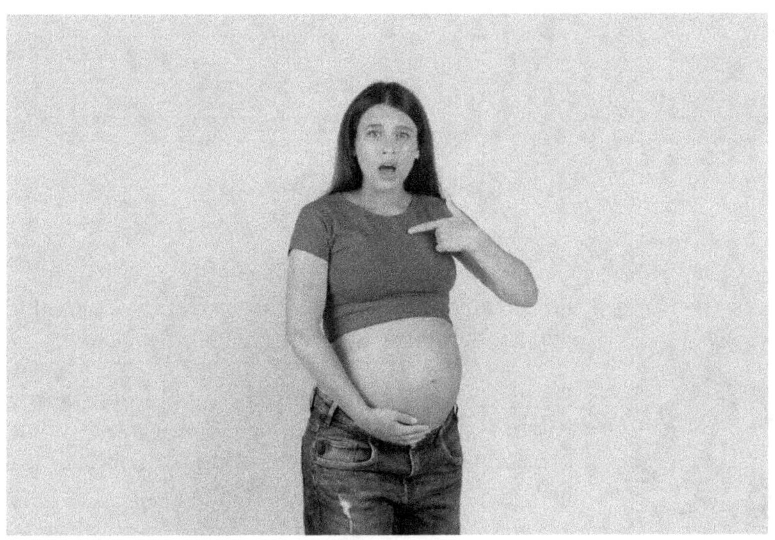

his book was designed to cover as much info as possible but I know I have probably issed something, or some new amazing discovery that has just come out.

 you notice something missing or have a question that I failed to answer, please get in uch and let me know. If I can, I will email you an answer and also update the book so hers can also benefit from it.

hanks For Being Awesome :)

Submit Your Questions / Comments At:
Get In Touch Babydreamers.net

Get How To Be A Super Mom 100% FREE

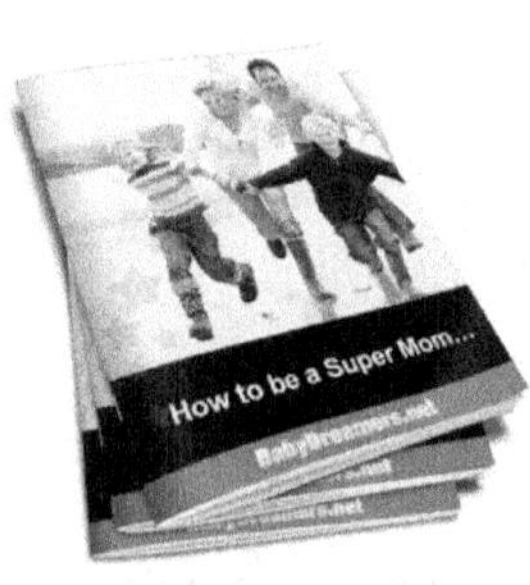

For being one of our amazing readers, we would love to offer you another book we have created, 100% free.

Being a mom is probably the most important job in the world – we've all heard that, and it's true. You're bringing up the next generation of wonderful, intelligent, loving, creative, responsible people.

We all want to be Super Mom and to be everything and do everything, but it this possible?

Being a Super Mom is possible, but you have to learn how to empower yourself to be the kind of Super Mom that you feel you need to be, keeping in mind that the title Super Mom doesn't mean the same thing to everyone.

Get How to be a Super Mom For Free